I0429928

INTEGRATIVE NUTRITION THERAPY

Revitalize Your Well-Being, A
Comprehensive Guide To Targeting Key
Issues, Focusing On Holistic Wellness,
And Embracing Nutritional Healing

DR. WANDA MENDENHALL

DISCLAIMER

This book is the result of the author's own expertise, insight, and experience in the area of treatment. The author has no affiliation with any particular firm, business, or person mentioned in this article. The content in this book is based exclusively on the author's knowledge and should not be construed as professional advice or a replacement for professional treatment or counseling.

Readers are recommended to seek professional counsel or guidance based on their unique circumstances or requirements. The author and publisher are not liable for any actions done in reliance on the information included in this book. Every person's circumstance is unique, so what works for one person may not work for another.

This book attempts to provide insights and knowledge for both education and personal growth.

The author does not recommend any certain therapy strategy or practice over another. Readers should exercise caution and check with trained specialists before using any knowledge or strategies discussed in this book.

By reading this book, the reader understands and accepts that the author and publisher are not accountable for any direct or indirect repercussions, damages, or losses that occur from the use or misuse of the material included herein.

Table of Contents

CHAPTER ONE

Introduction

Nutrition is critical to sustaining health and avoiding illness. Nutrition treatment has changed throughout time, covering numerous concepts and approaches. Integrative Nutrition Therapy (INT) is a practice that combines traditional, holistic, and contemporary approaches to nutrition, emphasizing a thorough knowledge of diet's influence on health and well-being.

This multifaceted approach incorporates many techniques to maximize dietary treatments for those seeking improved health outcomes.

Integrative Nutrition Therapy is based on a holistic paradigm that recognizes the interdependence of multiple aspects of health, such as physical, mental, emotional, and even spiritual components.

It integrates traditional nutritional research with complementary and alternative techniques, taking into account the individuality of each person's biochemistry, lifestyle, and tastes.

The emphasis is not only on food and nutrition, but also on lifestyle changes, mind-body approaches, and individualized treatments to address health difficulties.

Historical Perspectives On Nutrition And Health

Since ancient times, people have understood the link between diet and health. Food's importance in supporting health was chronicled in historical literature from civilizations such as ancient Greece, Egypt, and China.

The formalization of nutrition research, however, started in the nineteenth century, with discoveries such as the discovery of vitamins and macronutrients. As knowledge advanced, the emphasis switched from correcting vitamin shortages to comprehending the role of food in chronic illnesses such as cardiovascular disease, diabetes, and obesity.

Evolution Of Integrative Approaches In Nutrition

The limitations of traditional techniques prompted the emergence of Integrative Nutrition Therapy. While classical nutrition research produced useful insights, it often ignored individual differences in response to food and lifestyle. As a reaction to this gap, integrative techniques arose, recognizing that a "one-size-fits-all" paradigm may not meet everyone's requirements. To provide a more individualized and complete approach to nutrition and health, this progression includes components from traditional medicine, holistic practices such as Ayurveda and Traditional Chinese Medicine, and current scientific research.

Integrative Nutrition Therapy has entered the mainstream in recent decades, thanks to a growing amount of data confirming the effectiveness of integrative therapies and greater consumer interest in holistic health. It is now acknowledged as a beneficial supplement to traditional healthcare, providing a more individualized, patient-centered approach that attempts to promote general well-being as well as treat ailments.

Integrating evidence-based nutrition research with complementary approaches encourages people to take an active part in their health journey, creating a greater awareness of the complex link between nutrition, lifestyle, and well-being.

CHAPTER TWO

Foundations Of Integrative Nutrition

Integrative Nutrition is based on a broad understanding that recognizes the individuality of each person. It takes into account different nutritional philosophies, cultural variances, and the influence of lifestyle variables on health.

This method takes into account not just the nutrients in food, but also the food's quality, how it's grown or produced, and its possible impacts on the body beyond simply nourishment.

It also highlights the significance of treating the mind-body link, acknowledging the influence of stress, emotional well-being, and mental health on food habits and overall health results. The underlying idea is that health is more than just the absence of sickness; it is about reaching optimum physical, mental, and emotional well-being via eating.

Nutritional Biochemistry And Metabolism

The study of how nutrients in a diet interact inside the body, influencing numerous physiological processes, is known as nutritional biochemistry. This area of study looks at how macronutrients (carbohydrates, proteins, and fats) and micronutrients (vitamins and minerals) are absorbed, digested, and used to sustain health.

Metabolism, on the other hand, refers to the intricate network of biochemical events that take place inside cells to transform foods into energy, cell building blocks, and other vital substances necessary for body functioning. Understanding these processes is critical in integrative nutrition because it allows you to personalize dietary recommendations based on your particular metabolic demands, health objectives, and possible health issues.

Holistic Understanding Of Food And Nutrition

When it comes to food and nutrition, Integrative Nutrition stresses the need for a holistic approach.

It understands that food is more than simply a source of calories; it's also information that interacts with our genes, controls our hormones, and affects our general health. This strategy takes into account not just the nutritional content of food, but also its quality, origin, cooking techniques, and the individual's connection with food.

It also includes the cultural, emotional, and social components of eating, recognizing that our food choices are impacted by reasons other than fundamental nutritional demands. Integrative nutritionists strive to encourage mindful eating by adopting a holistic approach, assisting clients in developing a healthy connection with food, and making educated decisions that feed both body and mind.

Role Of Micronutrients In Integrative Nutrition

Despite being needed in lesser amounts than macronutrients, micronutrients—vitamins and minerals—are important for a variety of physiological activities. These micronutrients are important in integrative nutrition because they influence activities such as immunological function, energy generation, enzyme activity, and cell maintenance.

Integrative nutritionists analyze an individual's micronutrient status using a variety of methodologies, taking into account aspects such as absorption, use, and excretion. This individualized approach enables focused therapies, such as dietary changes or supplements, to address particular deficiencies or imbalances that may influence an individual's well-being.

To summarize, Integrative Nutrition Therapy is a multidimensional strategy that combines several disciplines to comprehend the complicated link between food, nutrition, and health. It analyzes an individual's particular demands, lifestyle, and biological composition, to optimize health and well-being via tailored and holistic techniques.

CHAPTER THREE

Integrative Nutrition Assessment

Integrative Nutrition Assessment is a comprehensive way of assessing a person's nutritional status that takes into account not just conventional areas of nutrition but also a larger viewpoint that encompasses lifestyle, heredity, environment, and general well-being.

This approach acknowledges that each individual is unique and that their nutritional requirements are impacted by a variety of variables other than the fundamental nutrients.

Traditional Vs. Integrative Assessment Methods

Traditional nutrition evaluation approaches often emphasize measurable data such as calorie consumption, macronutrient and micronutrient levels, and anthropometric measures. While these measurements are useful, they only give a partial picture of an individual's nutritional state.

Integrative evaluation approaches go beyond typical measures by including a more in-depth study. This involves evaluating the person's lifestyle, stress levels, sleep habits, intestinal health, and any environmental exposures. Integrative techniques also take into account the mind-body link, acknowledging the influence of mental and emotional well-being on nutritional health.

Functional Nutrition Assessment

The Functional Nutrition Assessment is an important part of integrative nutrition. It entails recognizing imbalances or dysfunctions in the physiological processes of the body and comprehending how these imbalances lead to health problems.

This approach sees the body as an interrelated system and attempts to address the underlying causes of nutritional issues rather than just treating symptoms.

Functional Nutrition Assessment may include measuring hormone levels, immunological function, gut health, and inflammatory markers. Practitioners may build focused therapies to help the body reach optimum function and balance by recognizing underlying abnormalities.

Integrating Personalized Health Data

Personalized health data is critical in assessing integrative nutrition. This entails gathering and evaluating data particular to an individual, taking into account aspects such as genetics, epigenetics, metabolic function, and personal health history. This individualized data enables practitioners to adjust dietary advice to each individual's specific requirements.

Technological advances, such as genetic testing and wearable gadgets, give vital insights about a person's health profile. The incorporation of this individual data enables a more detailed assessment of nutritional needs, possible sensitivities, and recommended dietary practices.

Finally, Integrative Nutrition evaluation offers a paradigm leap in the area of nutrition, transcending the constraints of standard evaluation methodologies. Practitioners may better lead people toward optimum health and well-being by adopting a holistic approach that acknowledges uniqueness and includes individualized health data. This integrated approach is consistent with the view that nutrition is a dynamic and customized part of total health, rather than a one-size-fits-all paradigm.

CHAPTER FOUR

The Gut-Brain Connection

The bidirectional contact between the gastrointestinal (GI) tract and the brain is referred to as the gut-brain connection. This complex interaction is critical to preserving general health and well-being. Communication takes place via a variety of channels, including the neurological system, immunological system, and endocrine system.

The enteric nervous system (ENS), sometimes known as the "second brain," is a complex network of neurons implanted in the intestinal lining. This system interacts with the CNS, regulating activities including digestion, food absorption, and immunological responses. The brain, on the other hand, transmits signals to the stomach that influence motility, secretion, and the makeup of the gut microbiota.

Disruptions in the gut-brain axis have been related to a variety of health issues, including gastrointestinal illnesses such as IBS and IBD, as well as neurological disorders such as anxiety, depression, and even neurodegenerative diseases such as Alzheimer's.

Gut Microbiota And Its Impact On Health

The gut microbiota, a varied collection of microorganisms found in the GI tract, is critical to maintaining a healthy gut-brain axis. The microbiota is made up of bacteria, viruses, fungi, and other microorganisms that work together to aid digestion, nutrient absorption, and immunological function.

The balance of the gut microbiota is critical for health since an imbalance (dysbiosis) may cause a variety of health problems. Obesity, autoimmune illnesses, and mental health difficulties have all been linked to dysbiosis. Metabolites produced by the gut microbiota, such as short-chain fatty acids (SCFAs), impact both local and systemic physiological processes.

Dietary changes, prebiotics, and probiotics are often used to improve gut health. These are intended to encourage the development of beneficial bacteria, increase microbial diversity, and contribute to a healthy gut environment.

Neurotransmitters And Cognitive Function

Neurotransmitters are chemical messengers that send messages from nerve cells (neurons) in the brain to other sections of the nervous system. Serotonin, dopamine, and gamma-aminobutyric acid (GABA) are among the neurotransmitters produced and stored in the stomach.

Serotonin, sometimes known as the "feel-good" neurotransmitter, is essential for mood, hunger, and sleep regulation. The fact that the stomach produces 90% of serotonin emphasizes the relevance of gut health in mental wellness. Neurotransmitter imbalances have been related to illnesses such as depression, anxiety, and cognitive deterioration.

The gut-brain axis also regulates neurotransmitter production and availability in the brain. As a result, keeping a healthy stomach may improve cognitive performance and emotional well-being.

Strategies For Gut-Brain Optimization

1. **Dietary Interventions:** A fiber-rich, prebiotic- and probiotic-rich diet promotes a varied and healthy gut flora. Beneficial bacteria may be introduced via fermented foods such as yogurt, kefir, and sauerkraut.

2. Chronic stress has a deleterious influence on the gut-brain axis. Meditation, yoga, and mindfulness are all practices that may help decrease stress and increase intestinal health.

3. Physical exercise has been proven to impact the gut flora and stimulate the release of neurotransmitters linked to

enhanced mood and cognitive performance.

4. Probiotic Supplements: Probiotic supplements may be advantageous in certain circumstances, particularly following antibiotic therapy or in illnesses linked with dysbiosis.

5. Individual differences in gut microbiota composition and dietary reactions must be recognized in personalized nutrition. Individual dietary recommendations may be optimized by personalized nutrition, which is influenced by variables such as genetics and gut microbiota study.

To summarize, understanding and managing the gut-brain link is a comprehensive strategy for promoting overall health that includes both physical and mental well-being. Integrative nutrition treatment, which takes into account the interaction of the gut, food, and brain function, may have dramatic and beneficial impacts on an individual's health.

CHAPTER FIVE

Therapeutic Diets In Integrative Nutrition

Therapeutic diets are important in Integrative Nutrition Therapy because they concentrate on utilizing food to enhance health and treat particular health issues. These diets are adjusted to individual requirements, taking allergies, intolerances, illnesses, and general health objectives into account.

The method includes a variety of dietary treatments, including elimination diets, gut-healing protocols, and protocols addressing particular health concerns such as diabetes, cardiovascular disease, autoimmune illnesses, and others.

These diets are not one-size-fits-all; rather, they are tailored to an individual's biochemistry, health issues, and nutritional needs. To promote the body's healing and maintenance processes, they often entail the exclusion or inclusion of particular food categories, vitamin supplementation, and a concentration of complete, nutrient-dense meals.

Anti-Inflammatory Diets

Chronic inflammation has been related to several health problems, including autoimmune illnesses, heart disease, diabetes, and even certain malignancies. Anti-inflammatory diets try to reduce inflammation by prioritizing anti-inflammatory meals while limiting or eliminating those that cause inflammatory reactions.

These diets often contain an abundance of fruits, vegetables, whole grains, healthy fats (such as those found in avocados, almonds, and olive oil), fatty fish high in omega-3 fatty acids, and anti-inflammatory spices such as turmeric and ginger. They often restrict or eliminate processed meals, sugar, trans fats, and refined carbs, all of which may lead to inflammation.

Metabolic Typing And Personalized Diets

Metabolic typing is based on the idea that each person has a unique metabolic process, and hence their nutritional demands differ correspondingly. This method acknowledges that individuals metabolize nutrients differently depending on variables such as heredity, lifestyle, and environment. Personalized diets may be devised to maximize energy levels, weight control, and general health by recognizing an individual's metabolic type.

Some people, for example, may benefit from a higher protein, lower carbohydrate diet, whilst others may benefit from a more balanced macronutrient ratio. Understanding these distinctions allows diets to be tailored to an individual's metabolic demands.

Plant-Based Nutrition Approaches

Plant-based nutrition advocates a diet high in plant-derived foods such as fruits, vegetables, whole grains, nuts, seeds, and legumes. This method improves health by offering an abundance of vitamins, minerals, antioxidants, and fiber while limiting the use of processed foods and animal products.

Plant-based diets have been linked to a variety of health advantages, including a decreased risk of heart disease, lower blood pressure, better weight management, and improved blood sugar control. They may also help to ensure environmental sustainability by lowering the environmental impact of animal husbandry.

Integrative Nutrition Therapy embraces these varied dietary methods, acknowledging their significance and advocating for a tailored, holistic approach to health and nutrition. Practitioners may assist clients with dietary practices that improve general well-being and treat particular health conditions by taking into account individual requirements, preferences, and health objectives.

CHAPTER SIX

Integrative Nutrition And Chronic Diseases

Integrative nutrition understands that food has a significant influence on chronic illnesses. To prevent and manage these illnesses, it stresses the use of complete foods, nutrients, and lifestyle changes. Individualized treatment is emphasized, with genetic predispositions, environmental circumstances, and personal health history all taken into account.

Diabetes And Blood Sugar Regulation

To manage blood sugar levels, INT recommends a balanced diet rich in fiber, low-glycemic index foods, and healthy fats. It also promotes mindful eating, portion management, and physical exercise regularly.

Vitamins and herbs: Some integrative techniques include vitamins like chromium and alpha-lipoic acid, as well as plants like cinnamon and bitter melon, which are thought to help with blood sugar management.

Stress Management: Stress affects blood sugar levels. Mindfulness, meditation, and yoga are key components of INT for stress management and, as a result, improved blood sugar control.

INT promotes a heart-healthy diet rich in fruits, vegetables, whole grains, lean meats, and healthy fats such as omega-3 fatty acids. It also advises less processed meals, salt, and trans fats.

Supplements: Omega-3 fatty acids, Coenzyme Q10, and magnesium are often prescribed in INT to improve heart health and prevent inflammation.

To enhance cardiovascular health, INT focuses a strong emphasis on lifestyle modifications such as smoking cessation, stress management strategies, regular exercise, and proper sleep.

Anti-Inflammatory Diet: INT advocates for an anti-inflammatory diet rich in antioxidants, omega-3 fatty acids, and probiotics. It also recommends avoiding possible trigger foods that may aggravate autoimmune reactions.

Gut Health: There is an emphasis on gut health since it is important in autoimmune disorders. Probiotics, prebiotics, and dietary changes are used to sustain a healthy gut microbiota.

Stress Reduction: Stress may cause or exacerbate autoimmune diseases. To control symptoms, INT incorporates stress-reduction practices such as meditation, yoga, and therapy.

Supplements and herbs: In integrative treatments, some supplements like vitamin D, turmeric, and probiotics are routinely advised to modify the immune system and decrease inflammation.

Integrative Nutrition Therapy is a holistic approach to chronic illness management. It strives to promote general health and well-being while addressing the unique requirements of persons with chronic diseases by stressing tailored diets, lifestyle changes, stress management, and the integration of complementary treatments. Individuals must, however, collaborate with skilled healthcare providers to develop individualized strategies that address their specific health needs.

CHAPTER SEVEN

Mindful Eating And Behavioral Strategies

Mindful Eating is a discipline that entails being completely present and engaged when eating. It is about paying attention to the sensory sensations, ideas, and emotions that accompany eating. Behavioral methods are critical in developing mindful eating habits. These tactics are as follows:

1. Encourage people to notice hunger and satiety indicators, comprehend emotional eating triggers, and recognize habitual eating habits.

2. Slow Eating: Emphasizing the significance of eating slowly, properly chewing food, and appreciating the flavors and textures. This permits the body to more appropriately sense fullness.

3. Reduce distractions (such as TV or phones) during meals and practice dining in a peaceful, relaxed atmosphere to create an environment favorable to mindful eating.

4. **Portion Control:** Educating people on proper portion sizes and how to serve oneself mindfully to prevent overeating.

Psychology Of Eating

The Psychology of Eating entails investigating the intricate interaction between food-related thoughts, emotions, and actions. This field investigates:

1. Understanding how emotions impact eating patterns is referred to as emotional eating. Different eating habits may be triggered by stress, boredom, melancholy, and happiness.

2. **Cognitive Behavioral Approaches:** The use of cognitive strategies to question and alter mental patterns about food, body image, and self-esteem.

3. Recognizing how psychological well-being affects digestion, nutrition absorption, and general health.

Mindful Eating Practices

Mindful eating practices are approaches that help people establish a mindful eating approach:

1. **Mindful Awareness:** Encouraging people to pay nonjudgmental attention to the present moment when eating, concentrating on sensory perceptions such as taste, smell, and texture.

2. **Mindful Meal Planning:** Emphasizing mindful meal selection and preparation, taking nutritional requirements and personal preferences into account.

3. Mindful Breathing: The practice of using breathing methods to center oneself before meals, so assisting in relaxation and attention.

Behavior Change Techniques In Nutrition Therapy

Behavior modification strategies are critical in assisting people in adopting and maintaining good eating habits:

1. Goal defining: Assisting people in defining realistic, attainable dietary goals to encourage motivation and commitment.

2. Self-monitoring: Encouraging people to keep track of their eating habits, thoughts, and feelings about food.

This aids in the identification of trends and areas for improvement.

3. Social Support: The use of social networks or support groups to give encouragement and accountability throughout the behavior change process.

Integrating mindful eating with behavioral tactics, comprehending the psychology of eating, practicing mindful eating practices, and using behavior modification approaches may result in a holistic approach to nutrition therapy, creating healthy connections with food and general well-being.

CHAPTER EIGHT

Integrative Nutrition And Physical Activity

Integrative nutrition stresses the importance of diet and exercise in reaching optimum health. It recognizes that a healthy diet and regular exercise are essential components of total well-being. Rather than seeing nutrition and physical exercise as distinct things, integrative nutrition acknowledges a symbiotic connection in which one complements and increases the advantages of the other.

Exercise Physiology And Nutrition

Exercise physiology is the study of how the body reacts to and adapts to physical exertion.

Nutrition is crucial in supporting these physiological functions. For example, macronutrients such as carbs, proteins, and fats supply energy that is required for exercise performance, but micronutrients such as vitamins and minerals support numerous physiological activities that are required during physical activity. Understanding the dietary requirements of the body about various kinds, intensities, and durations of exercise is critical for optimal performance and recovery.

Nutrient Timing For Performance

Nutrient timing refers to the strategic consumption of nutrients in connection to exercise sessions to promote performance, recuperation, and adaptation. Consuming macronutrients around exercises, such as carbs before exercise for energy or protein after exercise for muscle repair, may have a substantial influence on performance and recuperation. This idea emphasizes the significance of customizing diet to the body's metabolic and physiological needs during and after physical exercise.

Integrating Nutrition With Fitness Goals

Integrating nutrition with fitness goals entails developing tailored nutrition plans that are connected with particular fitness goals. A tailored nutrition plan is essential whether you want to lose weight, grow muscle, enhance your endurance, or improve your general fitness. Calorie intake, macronutrient distribution, hydration, and micronutrient assistance customized to individual requirements are all factors to consider. Integrating diet and exercise objectives also need ongoing evaluation and modification to achieve optimum development and long-term outcomes.

Essentially, combining diet and physical exercise is a dynamic and individualized strategy. It's not just about what one eats or how one exercises on their own, but about knowing how these components interact together to enhance health, performance, and general well-being. Integrative nutrition treatment recognizes this interaction by providing a complete framework that enables people to make educated decisions to attain their health and fitness goals.

CHAPTER NINE

Environmental And Ethical Considerations

Sustainable Nutrition Practices

Sustainable eating practices stress the consumption of foods produced in a way that has the least environmental effect. This entails:

1. **Locally Produced Foods:** Promoting the use of locally produced foods helps to lower the carbon footprint associated with transportation. It helps local economies and strengthens the bond between customers and producers.

2. Seasonal Eating: Choosing seasonal meals decreases the need for energy-intensive techniques of preserving out-of-season products. It also encourages dietary diversity.

3. Organic and Regenerative Agriculture: Promoting organic agricultural techniques reduces the need for synthetic pesticides and fertilizers, hence lowering soil and water pollution. Furthermore, campaigning for regenerative agriculture aids in the restoration of soil health and biodiversity.

Ethical Food Choices

Ethical concerns in food selection include a variety of aspects, including:

1. **Animal Welfare:** Promoting the consumption of animal products from sources that value the ethical treatment of animals, such as free-range or pasture-raised animal products, may encourage more humane agricultural techniques.

2. **Fair Trade and Social Responsibility:** Supporting fair trade programs guarantees that producers, particularly those in developing countries, are fairly compensated for their efforts. This method helps in the fight against food production exploitation.

3. **Reducing Food Waste:** It is critical to educate people about the environmental effects of food waste and to encourage

ways to reduce waste at all levels, from production to consumption.

Impact Of Food Production On The Environment

Food production has a big environmental impact:

1. Agriculture uses a substantial quantity of water, contributes to deforestation, and occupies enormous geographical areas. Sustainable approaches such as precision agriculture and water conservation are critical for mitigating this effect.

2. **Greenhouse Gas Emissions:** Livestock production, particularly on a large scale, contributes considerably to greenhouse gas emissions.

This effect may be mitigated by shifting to plant-based diets or limiting meat intake.

3. Biodiversity Loss: Monoculture and intensive agricultural techniques may result in biodiversity loss. Diverse cropping systems and agroecological techniques aid in the preservation of ecosystems and their functions.

Integrative nutrition treatment includes these factors by teaching people about the interdependence of food, health, and the environment. It encourages a holistic approach to food intake that not only feeds the body but also adheres to ethical ideals and reduces environmental impact.

Integrative nutrition treatment may greatly improve personal health and the well-being of the world by encouraging awareness of food choices, promoting sustainable habits, and advocating for ethical choices.

CHAPTER TEN

Future Directions In Integrative Nutrition

Integrative Nutrition is an interdisciplinary discipline that combines traditional wisdom with current research to promote overall health. Looking forward, many paths seem promising:

1. **Precision Nutrition:** Technological advancements provide individualized nutritional recommendations based on a person's genetic composition, microbiota, lifestyle, and health state. Precision Nutrition seeks to personalize nutritional guidance to an individual's exact requirements.

2. Nutrigenomics and Nutrigenetics: These fields study how nutrients interact with genes and how genetic variants influence dietary responses. This area has the potential to have a considerable influence on individualized nutrition, illness prevention, and management.

3. Functional Foods and Nutraceuticals: Researchers are working to create functional foods that are rich in bioactive chemicals and provide health advantages that go beyond basic nutrition. Nutraceuticals, which include supplements and fortified meals, may play an important role in preventative healthcare.

4. Wearable Technology and Digital Health: The integration of digital tools and wearable devices allows for real-time monitoring of nutritional intake, physical activity, and health markers. This information may be used to create tailored dietary recommendations and promote healthy behaviors.

Integrative Nutrition Research And Innovations

1. Understanding the intricate interplay between the gut flora and diet offers enormous promise for controlling numerous health issues and enhancing general well-being.

2. Plant-Based Diets and Sustainable Nutrition: As concerns about health, environmental sustainability, and animal welfare rise, so does research into plant-based diets and sustainable food production techniques.

3. Exploring the delicate link between mental health, emotional well-being, and eating habits is gaining popularity. Integrating mental health and dietary strategies might reshape holistic well-being.

Shaping The Future Of Personalized Nutrition

1. Big Data Integration: By combining huge information from diverse sources, such as genetics, microbiomics, and lifestyle variables, tailored nutrition recommendations will be refined.

2. Education and Accessibility: Promoting nutritional literacy and making tailored nutrition available to a broad range of groups will be critical to obtaining widespread health benefits.

3. Collaboration and interdisciplinary approaches will stimulate innovation and the use of customized nutrition in healthcare by bridging barriers across disciplines such as nutrition, medicine, technology, and psychology.

To summarize, the future of integrative nutrition has enormous potential, driven by technology improvements, new research, and a focus on tailored methods to empower people to optimize their health and well-being.

Conclusion

Integrative Nutrition Therapy results in a holistic approach to well-being that recognizes the complicated links between diet, lifestyle, and health. It highlights the customized character of nutrition in its conclusion, acknowledging that there is no one-size-fits-all approach. Rather, it argues for a more personalized approach that takes into account not just the nutritional worth of food but also cultural, emotional, and psychological factors.

The conclusion emphasizes the importance of eating a well-balanced diet that feeds the body while also supporting mental and emotional well-being. It emphasizes the value of whole, unprocessed foods, mindful eating, and the function of food as medicine. It also recognizes that this journey is about more than just what's on the plate; it also includes stress management, physical exercise, and a supportive atmosphere to promote overall health.

In addition, the conclusion of Integrative Nutrition Therapy emphasizes the need for continued research and teaching. The area is dynamic, growing with new nutritional science discoveries, and it highlights the significance of remaining current with the newest research to optimize therapy methods.

Finally, the conclusion praises people's ability to take responsibility for their health via educated decisions, resulting in a harmonious balance between nutrition, wellness, and lifestyle for a satisfying and vibrant existence.

THE END